Short Wordless Picture Bo

This collection of short wordless picture books
speech, language and communication needs a.
sentence and narrative skills through storytelling. Each book is comprised of six
colourful images that follow a simple everyday routine such as 'Brushing Teeth',
'Having a Haircut' and 'Walking the Dog'. Unlike traditional picture books, they
follow a film scroll effect, showing the progression of time and allowing the
child to follow the story to its resolution. Because of their simplicity, the books
can support children as they move from simple to intermediate sentence levels,
as well as encouraging them to consider additional elements of language such
as cause and effect, sequencing and inference.

This resource includes:

- Ten beautifully illustrated picture books, each following a simple pattern of
  routine, disruption and resolution

- An accompanying guidebook including story scripts, cue questions and
  prompts for using the resource to support additional skills

Although developed specifically to help children with speech, language and
communication needs, this set is suitable for any child who requires support
and practice in developing their speech. It is an invaluable resource for speech
and language therapists, teaching staff and caregivers.

Kulvinder Kaur has received training in Applied Behavioural Analysis and
has taught children between the ages of 2 and 16 years for 15 years.
Her work has been mainly 1:1 with both verbal and non-verbal children.
The Applied Behavioural Analysis curriculum covers mainly language,
communication, social, cognitive, functional and academic skills. She currently
works as a Team Lead on programmes, involving assessing skills, designing
targets, creating lesson plans as well as producing resources. Alongside her
role, Kulvinder continues to develop her practical teaching skills by educating
children with a diagnosis of autism in mainstream primary schools and in
private practice, which has involved working with behavioural analysts, speech
and language therapists and multidisciplinary teams. She is the author of
Wordless Picture Books and Guide, published by Speechmark in April 2016.

Short Wordless Picture Books

Developing Sentence and Narrative Skills for People with Speech, Language and Communication Needs

Kulvinder Kaur

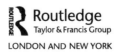

Routledge
Taylor & Francis Group

LONDON AND NEW YORK

First published 2020
by Routledge
2 Park Square, Milton Park, Abingdon, Oxon OX14 4RN

and by Routledge
52 Vanderbilt Avenue, New York, NY 10017

Routledge is an imprint of the Taylor & Francis Group, an informa business

© 2020 Kulvinder Kaur

British Library Cataloguing-in-Publication Data
A catalogue record for this book is available from the British Library

Library of Congress Cataloging-in-Publication Data
Names: Kaur, Kulvinder, author.
Title: Short wordless picture books and guide : developing sentence and narrative skills for people with
    speech, language and communication needs / Kulvinder Kaur.
Description: Abingdon, Oxon ; New York : Routledge, 2020. | Includes bibliographical references. | Summary:
    "This collection of short wordless picture books helps to support children with speech, language and
    communication needs as they develop their expressive sentence and narrative skills through storytelling.
    Each book is comprised of six colourful images that follow a simple everyday routine such as 'Brushing
    Teeth', 'Having a Haircut' and 'Walking the Dog'. Unlike traditional picture books, they follow a film scroll
    effect, showing the progression of time and allowing the child to follow the story to its resolution. Because
    of their simplicity, the books can support children as they move from simple to intermediate sentence
    levels, as well as encouraging them to consider additional elements of language such as cause and effect,
    sequencing and inference. This resource includes: - Ten beautifully illustrated picture books, each following
    a simple pattern of routine, disruption and resolution - An accompanying guidebook including story scripts,
    cue questions and prompts for using the resource to support additional skills Although developed
    specifically to help children with speech, language and communication needs, this set is suitable for any
    child who requires support and practice in developing their speech. It is an invaluable resource for speech
    and language therapists, teaching staff and caregivers"— Provided by publisher.
Identifiers: LCCN 2019017114 | ISBN 9781138477575 (paperback) | ISBN 9781351104364 (ebook)
Subjects: LCSH: Picture books for children—Educational aspects. | Stories without words. |
    Communicative disorders in children. | Speech disorders—Education. | Language arts. | Children
    with disabilities—Communication.
Classification: LCC LB1044.9.P49 .K38 2020 | DDC 371.33—dc23
LC record available at https://lccn.loc.gov/2019017114

ISBN: 978-0-367-34013-1 (pbk)
ISBN: 978-1-138-47757-5 (set pbk)
ISBN: 978-1-351-10436-4 (set ebk)

Typeset in Lato
by Apex CoVantage, LLC

Visit the eResources: www.routledge.com/9781138477575

Pack contents

Guidebook

Making Cereal

Going to School

Brushing Teeth

Having a Haircut

Walking the Dog

In the Bakery

In the Park

Playing Hide and Seek

At School

Swimming

User Guide contents

Chapter 1 Introduction 1

Chapter 2 How to use this resource 3

Chapter 3 Story scripts: Simple to intermediate 9

Chapter 4 Additional skills 17

    WH questions. 17

    Recognising emotions and situation-based emotions. 19

    Cause and effect. 24

    Sequencing 28

    Time concepts. 31

        Connectives 32

        Pronouns. 32

    Inference 33

    Topical conversation. 42

    Further reading 44

Chapter 1 Introduction

This series of wordless picture books aims to help children with speech, language and communication needs (SLCN) develop their expressive sentence and narrative skills through learning to tell stories. The resource is appropriate for children aged three onwards and is aimed at any child from this age who requires practice in developing their speech and who may be receiving speech and language therapy input. The stories are an aid for speech and language therapists, learning support and teaching assistants, teachers, caregivers and parents.

The resource comprises ten simple stories and the sentence levels can be advanced from simple to intermediate. They can be told by children who are starting to form simple sentences and children who require help with forming grammatically correct, longer and more descriptive sentences.

The stories have been intentionally developed around themes that are likely to be familiar to children, and they follow a film scroll effect; this formula has been used to facilitate understanding for children with limited receptive language. General story and picture books do not follow this formula and therefore are not always appropriate to use because of the unfamiliarity of events, ideas and language, and because the illustrations are often there to accompany the text and may 'jump' from one scene to another.

The formula of each story is a disruption or an interesting event in a familiar routine followed by a resolution. This guide offers strategies on how to teach and progress the child through each level and provides simple and intermediate scripts for each story. It has an additional skills section at the end to help develop key skills and comprehension

(Chapter 4). It is advisable to read Chapter 2, on teaching strategies, before progressing to Chapters 3 and 4.

Although this resource is primarily for SLCN, it can be used for literacy development by teachers in Early Years, Key Stage 1, and English Speakers of Other Languages.

Chapter 2　How to use this reSource

Who it's for

This resource is appropriate for children who have the following skills:

- have a repertoire of common receptive and expressive nouns, verbs, adjectives and prepositions
- able to recognise the above in pictures
- able to imitate three-word sentences, e.g., if you say to the child, 'Say "I want chips"', the child must be able to repeat.

Which stage to start from

The stories are divided in two sections based on the two sentence levels: simple and intermediate. Below is a table outlining what each sentence level consists of to help you decide which is the most appropriate for the child to start at:

	Description	Average words for each sentence / page	Average words for each story
Simple	This level mainly includes one clause: subject–verb–noun.	5 words	30 words
Intermediate	This level includes longer sentences which mainly consist of two joining clauses, and sometimes two one-clause sentences for a page. The sentences describe the story in more detail, and conjunctions are used to join the events on the page together and are sometimes used to join the events across pages together.	9 words	55 words

Start at the child's current word utterance level. If you're unsure of this, assess their level by asking them to say a four-word sentence and see if they can repeat it easily. If they can't, then start with simple sentences. If they can do simple sentences easily and can copy an eight-word sentence, start with the intermediate level.

How much to do at one time

This depends on a number of factors and will depend on each child and their individual progress.

In particular, the factors to consider are the child's attention to the task, their interest in the task, and the repetitions required for them to acquire the skills. Some may need to work on one book and one page at a time, while others may be able to work through a few pages and even a book at a time. It's important to be aware of the child's level and to work from that. So, if the child requires time to learn to put one four-word sentence together, then work on establishing this. Over time they will become more skilled at the task and you will be able to work through more.

If you only work through a page or two to begin with, you could tell the rest of the story to the child to expose them to the language.

How often

This also depends on the individual child and their rate of progress. The child may require more practice to retain the new skills in a lesson and over time.

When to move on to the next level

The aim is to teach the child the skill to the point of independence. Once they can independently tell the stories at their current level without support, then you can start making progress on the next level.

Teaching strategies

In this section there is a list of strategies to help the child learn. Some may be more helpful than others.

Verbal aids

- The first strategy to use is to tell the child the sentence, ask them to repeat it to you, and then work on them saying it independently.

- If they miss words from the sentence, say the sentence again but this time emphasise the missing word by saying it more clearly and slowly. For example, if the sentence is 'The boy is crying' and the child misses the word 'is', then say 'The boy iisss crying' and see if this helps the child to repeat the sentence back with the missing word.

- Split the sentence into two or more chunks. For example 1) The boy 2) is crying. Work on the first part and then move on to the second. Once the child can say the two separate parts, put them together.

- Tell the child the sentence, but pause at the word they tend to miss. They are expected to fill in that word. Prompt them to say it if you have to. After practice, check if they are then able to say the whole sentence with the missing word.

Visual aid

- Use a number strip to help the child fill in the missing word. Each number represents a word in the sentence. For example:

1	2	3	4
The	boy	is	crying.

Don't have the words under the numbers. Show the child that each number represents a word by pointing to each number as you say each word from the sentence. Ask the child to point with you and say each word. Once you have practised this together, get the child to use the number strip themselves. If they miss a word, stop them as they are doing it to ensure they say the word. Once they are able to say the sentence with the strip independently, check to see if they can say the sentence without it. For words that the child tends to miss, it may be helpful if you say the sentence and pause at the word's number, so that the child has to fill in that word.

Written aids

- It can be helpful to write the word/s that the child finds difficult to say on pieces of paper and, as they say the sentence, point to each word they have to remember to add when it's time to say it. Practise this together and then get them to do it independently. After they can do this independently a number of times, remove the words and see if they can remember to say the word without the written aid.

- You can write the full sentence down so that all the words are visible. Get the child to read it and then cover the beginning words they find easy to remember and slowly cover each one until you can cover up the whole sentence.

- Alternatively, write down the sentence and get the child to practise it. Then take it away and write it down as the child says it. If they get the sentence wrong, tell them the answer and re-do that part of the sentence. Practise this until the child can say the whole sentence independently.

Checking comprehension

If you are uncertain whether the child understands what's happening in the picture and the overall story, tell them the story and ask questions about it (see 'WH questions', Chapter 4, page 17).

If there is a particular part of a story that you think they do not understand, then it may be helpful to demonstrate this in person and explain, and then ask them 'What happened?' or 'What did I do?' Once you are sure the child understands, transfer this understanding to the story by retelling that part of it and asking them what the character is doing and/or what's happening.

Chapter 3 Section 1 Story Scripts

Levels: Simple to intermediate

Simple (29 words)

Book 1 Making Cereal

1   The girl pours the cereal

2   She pours milk on the table

3   She sees the mess

4   She wipes the table

5   She pours milk in the bowl

6   She eats the cereal

Intermediate (52 words)

Book 1 Making Cereal

1   The sleepy girl pours cereal in the bowl

2   Then she accidentally pours milk on the table

3   She is shocked to see the milk on the table

4   Next, she wipes the table with a cloth

5   After that, she pours the milk in the bowl

6   Last, she eats her cereal with a blue spoon

Simple (29 words)
Book 2 Going to School

1   The boy puts his shoes on

2   He puts his jacket on

3   He gets his bag

4   He opens the front door. It's raining

5   He gets an umbrella

6   He goes outside

Intermediate (51 words)
Book 2 Going to School

1   First, the boy puts his black school shoes on

2   Afterwards, he puts on his red jacket

3   Then he reaches for his blue school bag

4   He opens the front door and it's raining

5   So, he gets a yellow umbrella from the basket

6   Last, he holds up the umbrella and leaves his house

Simple (29 words)
Book 3 Brushing Teeth

1   The boy gets the toothpaste

2   He squeezes the toothpaste

3   It squirts on his face!

4   He wipes his face

5   He squeezes the toothpaste on the toothbrush

6   He brushes his teeth

Intermediate (49 words)
Book 3 Brushing Teeth

1   First the boy gets a toothbrush and toothpaste

2   Then he squeezes the toothpaste towards his face

3   Oops! The toothpaste accidentally squirts on to his face!

4   The boy wipes the toothpaste off his face with a tissue

5   Next, he squeezes the toothpaste on the toothbrush

6   Last he brushes his teeth

Simple (28 words)
Book 4 Having a Haircut

1   The hairdresser puts the cape on the boy

2   He shaves his hair

3   He sprays water on

4   He cuts his hair

5   He combs his hair

6   His haircut is finished

Intermediate (52 words)
Book 4 Having a Haircut

1   First, the hairdresser puts the cape on the boy

2   Then he shaves the boy's hair with a razor

3   Next he sprays water on the boy's hair

4   Then he cuts his hair with scissors

5   Afterwards, he combs his hair. The boy is smiling

6   Last, the haircut is finished and the boy likes it

Simple (29 words)
Book 5 Walking the Dog

1   The girl walks her dog

2   She sees her friend

3   She presses the traffic light button

4   She waits for the green man

5   She crosses the road

6   She hugs her friend

Intermediate (61 words)
Book 5 Walking the Dog

1   First, the girl walks her dog down the road

2   Then she sees her friend and waves at him

3   She wants to cross the road so she presses the traffic light button

4   Then she waits for the green man before crossing

5   When she sees the green man, she crosses the road

6   She gets to the other side and hugs her friend

Simple (30 words)

Book 6 In the Bakery

1   The girl wants a gingerbread man

2   The boy buys the gingerbread man

3   The girl cries

4   She chooses a pig biscuit

5   Her mum buys the biscuit

6   The girl eats the biscuit

Intermediate (54 words)

Book 6 In the Bakery

1   First, the girl points to the gingerbread man because she wants it

2   Then the boy buys the last gingerbread man

3   So the girl cries because she wanted it

4   Then she chooses to have a pig biscuit

5   Next the girl waits as her mum buys the biscuit

6   Then the girl happily eats the pig biscuit

Simple (31 words)

Book 7 In the Park

(The girl in the purple dress is called Mia and the girl in the pink dress is called Carmen)

1   The girls eat their ice creams

2   Mia drops her ice cream

3   She puts it in the bin

4   She cries

5   Carmen pushes her on the swing

6   Mia pushes Carmen on her swing

Intermediate (63 words)
Book 7 In the Park

1   First, the girls eat their ice creams while sitting on the swings

2   Mia drops her ice cream on the ground

3   So she picks it up and puts it in the bin

4   Then she cries because she doesn't have an ice cream

5   Carmen pushes her on the swing to make her feel better

6   Then Mia pushes Carmen on the swing. Mia is happy now

Simple (32 words)
Book 8 Playing Hide and Seek

1   The boy closes his eyes

2   The girl hides behind the curtain

3   The boy opens his eyes

4   He looks under the table

5   He looks behind the sofa

6   He finds her behind the curtain

Intermediate (59 words)
Book 8 Playing Hide and Seek

1   First, the boy closes his eyes and the girl goes to hide

2   Then he counts and she hides behind the curtain

3   Next, he finishes counting and opens his eyes

4   Then he looks under the table but she's not there

5   Then he looks behind the sofa but she's not there

6   Last he looks behind the curtain and he finds her

Simple (29 words)

Book 9 At School

(The girl on the left is called Julia and the girl on the right is called Tia)

1   The girls are working

2   Tia wants the felt pens

3   Julia gives them to her

4   They carry on working

5   The teacher comes to see

6   Tia shows the teacher her drawing

Intermediate (58 words)

Book 9 At School

1   First, Julia is writing and Tia is drawing at school

2   Then Tia asks Julia for the felt pens

3   So Julia gives the felt pens to her

4   Tia starts colouring her picture and Julia carries on with her writing

5   Then the teacher comes and looks at Julia's writing

6   Tia shows the teacher her drawing and the teacher likes it

Simple (34 words)

Book 10 Swimming

1   Dad puts armbands on the boy
2   Dad walks down the ladder
3   The boy is scared to go in the pool
4   He walks down the ladder
5   He starts swimming
6   He splashes water on his dad

Intermediate (56 words)

Book 10 Swimming

1   First, the boy's dad puts armbands on him
2   Then his dad walks down the ladder
3   The boy's dad asks the boy to get in but the boy is too scared
4   Then the boy walks down the ladder
5   Next, he starts to swim and his dad is happy
6   Last, the boy accidentally splashes water on his dad

Chapter 4 Additional skills

The books have been designed to enable practice and generalisation of a range of skills. This chapter covers these skills.

The skills in this section may need to be taught separately using skill-specific resources, and once the child has learnt them, they can be generalised with this resource. Some skills may be too advanced for the child at the time they are learning the stories; however, these can be worked on at a later point when the child is ready.

WH questions

The books have been designed to enable practice of simple and complex WH questions. Below are two tables with the range of simple and complex WH questions and ideas on some areas that can be covered for each WH question.

Start with the simple WH questions if the child requires work on these. Once they can do the simple ones confidently, move on to the complex questions, working on one at a time. Many of the complex questions will be covered in subsequent sections as they fall under other skills, so these can be worked on separately within these sections.

Simple WH questions

Who	Who is in the picture? Who is (doing)? Who is (feeling ...)? Who is on the ...?
What	What's on / in the ...? What are they doing? What are they wearing? What colour is? What are they feeling? What is it? What time of day is it?
Where	Where are they? Where are they going? Where are they looking? Where is the ...?
When	When did they (action)? Answer could be before or after, time of day / when something happened.

Complex WH questions

Why	Why are they feeling? Why are they (doing)? Why has ... happened?
What happened?	What happened? What happens next? What happened before? What do you think will happen next? What do you think happened before? What will happen if ...?
How	How did ... happen? How do you know ...?
What makes you think?	What makes you think that has happened? What makes you think ... is feeling this way? What makes you think that will happen next?

Recognising emotions and situation-based emotions

Each book covers two to three of the following main emotions: happy, sad, scared (worried), angry, shocked and surprised. The books can be used to practise identifying characters' emotions from their facial expressions. Simply ask the child how the character is feeling.

If a child is able to accurately label the emotions of characters, they can move on to explaining the reason for the characters' emotions. This can be worked on by asking them why the character is feeling that way. This will involve the child in explaining the situational cause of their emotion.

Below is a list of questions and answers you could use for the emotions and situation-based emotions in each book:

Questions and answers

Book 1 Making Cereal

	Questions	Answers
Page 1	How is the girl feeling?	Tired/sleepy
	Why is she feeling tired/sleepy?	Because it's the morning. She has just woken up.
Page 3	How is the girl feeling?	Shocked
	Why is she feeling shocked?	Because she accidentally poured milk on the table.
Page 6	How is the girl feeling?	Happy
	Why is she feeling happy?	Because she is eating her cereal.

Book 2 Going to School

	Questions	Answers
Page 4	How do you think the boy might be feeling?	Surprised
	Why might he be feeling surprised?	Because it's raining outside and he didn't know.

Book 3 Brushing Teeth

	Questions	Answers
Page 3	How is the boy feeling?	Shocked
	Why is he feeling shocked?	Because he accidentally squirted toothpaste on his face.

Book 4 Having a Haircut

	Questions	Answers
Page 1	How is the boy feeling?	Sad
	Why is he feeling sad?	Because he doesn't want to have a haircut.
Page 2	How is the boy feeling?	Scared
	Why is he feeling scared?	Because he doesn't like the razor.
Page 6	How is the boy feeling?	Happy
	Why is he feeling happy?	Because he likes his new haircut.

Book 5 Walking the Dog

	Questions	Answers
Page 1	How is the girl feeling?	Happy
	Why is she feeling happy?	Because she is walking her dog.
Page 2	How is the boy feeling?	Happy
	Why is he feeling happy?	Because he has seen his friend.
Page 6	How is the boy feeling?	Happy
	Why is he feeling happy?	Because he is hugging his friend.

Book 6 In the Bakery

	Questions	Answers
Page 3	How is the girl feeling?	Sad
	Why is she feeling sad?	Because she wanted the gingerbread man and the boy bought it.
	How is the boy feeling?	Happy
	Why is he happy?	Because he has bought a gingerbread man.
Page 5	How is the girl feeling?	Happy
	Why is she feeling happy?	Because she is getting a pig biscuit.
	How is the girl's mum feeling?	Happy
	Why is she feeling happy?	Because the girl is happy with her pig biscuit.

Book 7 In the Park

	Questions	Answers
Page 1	How are the girls feeling?	Happy
	Why are they feeling happy?	Because they are eating ice creams.
Page 2	How is Mia feeling?	Shocked
	Why is she feeling shocked?	Because she has dropped her ice cream.
Page 3 & 4	How is Mia feeling?	Sad
	Why is she feeling sad?	Because she dropped her ice cream.
Page 4	How is Carmen feeling?	Sad
	Why is she feeling sad?	Because Mia is crying/sad.
Page 5	How is Mia feeling?	Happy
	Why is she feeling happy?	Because Carmen is pushing her on the swing.
Page 6	How is Carmen feeling?	Happy
	Why is she feeling happy?	Because Mia is pushing her on the swing.

Book 8 Playing Hide and Seek

	Questions	Answers
Page 1, 2 & 3	How is the boy feeling?	Happy
	Why is he feeling happy?	Because he is playing hide and seek.
Page 6	How is the girl feeling?	Happy
	Why is she feeling happy?	Because the boy found her.
	How is the boy feeling?	Happy
	Why is he feeling happy?	Because he found the girl.

Book 9 At School

	Questions	Answers
Page 1	How are the girls feeling?	Happy
	Why are they feeling happy?	Because they are writing/drawing.
Page 5	How is the teacher feeling?	Happy
	Why is she feeling happy?	Because she likes the girl's writing.
	How is Julia feeling?	Happy
	Why is she feeling happy?	Because the teacher likes her writing.
Page 6	How is the teacher feeling?	Happy
	Why is she feeling happy?	Because she likes the girl's drawing.
	How is Tia feeling?	Happy
	Why is she feeling happy?	Because the teacher likes her drawing.

Book 10 Swimming

	Questions	Answers
Page 1	How are the boy and dad feeling?	Happy
	Why are they feeling happy?	Because they are about to swim.
Page 3	How is the boy feeling?	Scared
	Why is he feeling scared?	Because he is scared to go in the pool.

Book 10 Swimming (continued)

	Questions	Answers
Page 4	How is the boy's dad feeling?	Happy
	Why is he feeling happy?	Because the boy is going in the water.
Page 5	How is the boy's dad feeling?	Excited
	Why is he feeling excited?	Because the boy is swimming.
Page 6	How is the boy's dad feeling?	Surprised
	Why is he feeling surprised?	Because the boy is splashing him.

Cause and effect

In this section there are lists of questions and answers for helping the child understand and answer questions on cause and effect. These questions are to help them understand and explain what led to a result in aspects of the story. The previous section on situation-based emotions also falls under this skill. If the child has had difficulty understanding the story, working through these sections will help them make the links.

If the child is able to answer the questions on causes and effects, then you can work on whether they can predict the effect of a hypothetical cause. This skill will rely on them using their previous experience and knowledge of the world. Below are a couple of examples of this:

- For Book 1, you could ask: 'If there was no cereal left in the box, what could the girl do?'

- For Book 2, you could ask: 'If the basket did not have an umbrella in it, what could the boy do?'

Questions and answers

Book 1 Making Cereal

	Questions	Answers
Page 2	Why is the girl pouring milk on the table?	Because she is sleepy and not concentrating.
Page 2	Why is there milk on the table?	Because the girl poured it on the table.
Page 5	Why is there no milk on the table?	Because the girl cleaned it.

Book 2 Going to School

	Questions	Answers
Page 6	Why is the boy holding an umbrella?	Because it is raining.

Book 3 Brushing Teeth

	Questions	Answers
Page 3	Why is there toothpaste on the boy's face?	Because he squeezed it on his face.
Page 5	Why is there no toothpaste on the boy's face?	Because he wiped it off.

Book 4 Having a Haircut

	Questions	Answers
Page 3	Why is the boy's hair wet?	Because the hairdresser sprayed it with water.
Page 6	Why is the boy's hair shorter?	Because the hairdresser cut it.

Book 5 Walking the Dog

	Questions	Answers
Page 4	Why are they waiting by the traffic lights?	Because the traffic light is red.
Page 5	Why are they crossing the road?	Because the traffic light is green.

Book 6 In the Bakery

	Questions	Answers
Page 1	Why is the girl pointing at the gingerbread man?	Because she wants it.
Page 2	Why is the boy pointing at the gingerbread man?	Because he wants it.
Page 3	Why is the girl crying?	Because she wanted the gingerbread man but the boy took it.
Page 5	Why is the girl's mum buying the pig biscuit?	Because the girl wants it.

Book 7 In the Park

	Questions	Answers
Page 2	Why is the ice cream on the floor?	Because the girl dropped it.
Page 4	Why is Mia crying?	Because she dropped her ice cream on the floor.

Book 8 Playing Hide and Seek

	Questions	Answers
Page 3	Why can't you see the girl?	Because she is hiding behind the curtain.
Page 6	Why is the girl smiling?	Because the boy has found her.
Page 6	Why is the boy smiling?	Because he has found the girl.

Book 9 At School

	Questions	Answers
Page 3	Why is Fiona giving Tia the felt pens?	Because Fiona asked for them.
Page 6	Why does the teacher have her thumb up?	Because she likes Tia's drawing.

Book 10 Swimming

	Questions	Answers
Page 2	Why is the boy's dad going in the swimming pool?	To swim
Page 6	Why has the boy's dad put his hands up?	Because the boy is splashing him.

Sequencing

Sequencing can be done before or after the story has been introduced to the child. Working on this skill either way will involve the child using inference, problem solving and demonstrating the ability to order coherently. If the story has been introduced to the child, they will use their memory and understanding of the story.

Present the pictures to the child in a messy array and ask them to put the pictures in order. If the child is unsure of how to start, you could present them with the first picture, or first few, and ask them to complete the sequence. If the child is still unsure of the order, you could discuss the pictures first to help them identify what is happening in each picture which will help them problem solve.

If the child has read the story, you can work on their learning to sequence the events verbally. Ask them to recall the events in order and, once they have told a page of the story, place the picture of that page on the table. This is a good task for working on their memory and narrative skills.

There are five stages of sequencing that can be worked through:
Level 1 (2 step); **Level 2** (3 step) and **Level 3** (4 step)

Suggestions for which page combinations can be used for each book at all levels are outlined in the table below. Printouts of the picture cards for each story can be obtained from Speechmark's website at: www. routledge.com/9781138477575.

Book	Level 1: 2 step	Level 2: 3 step	Level 3: 4 step
Book 1 Making Cereal	Pages 1, 2 Pages 2, 3 Pages 3,4 Pages 5,6	Pages 1, 2, 3 Pages 1, 2, 4 Pages 2, 3, 4 Pages 1, 5, 6	Pages 1, 2, 3, 4 Pages 2, 3, 4, 5 Pages 3, 4, 5, 6
Book 2 Going to School	Pages 1, 2 Pages 2, 3 Pages 3, 4 Pages 4, 5 Pages 5, 6 Pages 4, 6	Pages 1, 2, 3 Pages 2, 3, 4 Pages 3, 4, 5 Pages 4, 5, 6 Pages 3, 4, 6	Pages 1, 2, 3, 4 Pages 2, 3, 4, 5 Pages 3, 4, 5, 6 Pages 1, 3, 4, 6
Book 3 Brushing Teeth	Pages 1, 2 Pages 2, 3 Pages 3, 4 Pages 5, 6 Pages 1, 6	Pages 1, 2, 3 Pages 2, 3, 4 Pages 1, 5, 6 Pages 1, 3, 4	Pages 1, 2, 3, 4 Pages 2, 3, 4, 5
Book 4 Having a Haircut	Pages 1, 2 Pages 1, 3 Pages 1, 4 Pages 4, 5 Pages 5, 6 Pages 4, 6	Pages 1, 4, 5 Pages 4, 5, 6 Pages 1, 4, 6 Pages 3, 4, 5 Pages 3, 4, 6	Pages 1, 3, 4, 5 Pages 1, 4, 5, 6 Pages 3, 4, 5, 6
Book 5 Walking the Dog	Pages 1, 2 Pages 2, 3 Pages 3, 4 Pages 4, 5 Pages 5, 6 Pages 2, 5	Pages 1, 2, 3 Pages 2, 3, 4 Pages 3, 4, 5 Pages 4, 5, 6 Pages 3, 5, 6 Pages 2, 3, 5	Pages 1, 2, 3, 4 Pages 1, 2, 3, 5 Pages 1, 2, 5, 6 Pages 2, 3, 4, 5 Pages 2, 3, 4, 6 Pages 2, 3, 5, 6 Pages 3, 4, 5, 6

Book	Level 1: 2 step	Level 2: 3 step	Level 3: 4 step
Book 6 In the Bakery	Pages 1, 2 Pages 2, 3 Pages 4, 5 Pages 5, 6 Pages 4, 6	Pages 1, 2, 3 Pages 2, 3, 4 Pages 4, 5, 6 Pages 2, 4, 5 Pages 2, 4, 6 Pages 2, 5, 6	Pages 1, 2, 3, 4 Pages 2, 4, 5, 6 Pages 1, 2, 4, 5 Pages 1, 2, 4, 6
Book 7 In the Park	Pages 1, 2 Pages 2, 3 Pages 2, 4	Pages 1, 2, 3 Pages 2, 3, 4 Pages 1, 2, 4	Pages 1, 2, 3, 4
Book 8 Playing Hide and Seek	Pages 1, 2 Pages 2, 3 Pages 2, 6	Pages 1, 2, 3 Pages 2, 3, 6	Pages 1, 2, 3, 4 Pages 1, 2, 3, 6 Pages 2, 3, 4, 6 Pages 2, 3, 5, 6
Book 9 At School	Pages 1, 2 Pages 2, 3 Pages 3, 4 Pages 4, 5 Pages 1, 4 Pages 2, 4 Pages 5, 6	Pages 1, 2, 3 Pages 2, 3, 4 Pages 2, 4, 5 Pages 4, 5, 6 Pages 1, 4, 5 Pages 1, 3, 4 Pages 1, 4, 6	Pages 1, 2, 3, 4 Pages 2, 3, 4, 5 Pages 3, 4, 5, 6 Pages 1, 4, 5, 6 Pages 1, 3, 4, 5 Pages 1, 3, 4, 6
Book 10 Swimming	Pages 1, 2 Pages 2, 3 Pages 3, 4 Pages 4, 5 Pages 5, 6 Pages 2, 4 Pages 1, 5 Pages 4, 6	Pages 1, 2, 3 Pages 2, 3, 4 Pages 3, 4, 5 Pages 4, 5, 6 Pages 1, 2, 4 Pages 1, 2, 5 Pages 1, 2, 6 Pages 2, 4, 5 Pages 2, 4, 6 Pages 3, 4, 6	Pages 1, 2, 3, 4 Pages 2, 3, 4, 5 Pages 2, 3, 4, 6 Pages 3, 4, 5, 6 Pages 1, 3, 4, 5 Pages 1, 3, 4, 6 Pages 2, 4, 5, 6

Time concepts

Key time concepts are:

- first
- then
- last
- now and next
- before and after.

Time concepts can be used as the child learns to tell the story and during sequencing. The child may need teaching to understand these concepts. Using a visual strategy is a good approach and this can be done by flicking through the book and pointing and moving your finger in the relevant direction as you teach each concept, or by using the sequence cards and laying out the pictures in order, and then moving your finger in the relevant direction as you teach each concept. You can ask the child to show you their understanding of these concepts by pointing (randomly) to what happens first, next, last etc. Once they are able to answer your time concept questions by showing you, they can work on being able to tell you the answer to these questions. Sometimes it can help to consolidate one concept before moving on to another. For example, teach 'after' first and, once the child has fully grasped this, teach 'before', and then work on them randomly. Once the concepts have been consolidated, you can work on generalising the language related to these concepts. Some examples are: end, beginning, start, finish, middle.

The teaching strategies in Chapter 2 give useful skills on how to help the child add the time concepts to their storytelling.

Connectives

The stories can be used to teach use of common connectives (and, but, so, because, when, who, etc). A few connectives have been added to the scripts, but you may choose to use the stories to develop this skill further. The teaching strategies in Chapter 2 offer ideas on how to teach them.

You could choose to teach connectives as 'words that help connect events together', and teach several connectives, so the child has a concept of the words they are adding and their purpose. As the connectives have their individual uses, to develop their understanding and help generalise, you could teach the child to apply the appropriate connective to a range of novel sentences.

Pronouns

Pronouns are integrated into the scripts; however, the books can be used to teach pronouns in a more focused way. The books can also be used to generalise work on pronouns. There is a good mix of male and female characters in the stories. If teaching for the first time, make sure the child can distinguish between boy and girl, and man and woman. Following this, teach that you say 'he', 'his' and 'him' for boys and men, and 'she', 'her' and 'hers' for girls and women. A visual chart representing this can help, if the child is able to read the words. Then ask the child to go through a story, or randomly through stories and pages, and label males as 'he' and females as 'she', and a group of people as 'they'. Once they can do this, they could integrate the pronoun into the sentences, e.g. '**She** is pointing to the gingerbread man.' Following this, you can start working on sentences that involve using possessive pronouns with the correct pronoun, for example '**He** is brushing **his** teeth.'

If the child has successfully applied these skills to all stories, then check they are able to generalise the language successfully to other contexts (real life events, other stories, TV shows).

Inference

In this section the child will learn to answer a question about a story and explain how they have come to the answer. They will be relying on what information the pictures give them. This could be: facts in the pictures; the emotions and desires of characters; relating to something that happened earlier on in the story; or an understanding based on the child's previous knowledge and experience. The following pages have a list of suggested questions and answers for working on this skill. The question 'How do you know?' is used but you could use and generalise to 'What makes you think that?', 'What do you think and why?' and 'How come you think that?'

You could also work on helping the child make **predictive inferences**, i.e. 'What is going to happen next?', and asking the child to explain why they think that will happen.

Questions and answers

Book 1 Making Cereal

	Questions	Answers
Page 1	What time of the day is it?	Morning
	How do you know?	Because the girl is having cereal and she is wearing her pyjamas.
	What room of the house is this?	The kitchen
	How do you know it's the kitchen?	Because I can see a fridge and a microwave, etc.
	How is the girl feeling?	Tired
	How do you know?	Because she is yawning.

Book 1 Making Cereal (continued)

	Questions	Answers
Page 2	Is the girl concentrating?	No
	How do you know?	Because she is pouring milk on the table.
Page 3	How is the girl feeling?	Shocked
	How do you know she is shocked?	Because her mouth and eyes are wide open.
Page 5	How is the girl feeling now?	Happy
	How do you know she is happy?	Because she is smiling.
	Is the girl still feeling tired?	No
	How do you know she is not tired?	Because her eyes are wide open.

Book 2 Going to School

	Questions	Answers
Page 1	Where is the boy going?	To school
	How do you know he is going to school?	Because he is wearing a school uniform.
	What time of the day do you think it is?	Morning
	How do you know it's the morning?	Because he is going to school.
	Do you think a woman and man live at the boy's house?	Yes
	How do you know they do?	Because I can see women's and men's shoes on the shoe rack.

Book 2 Going to School (continued)

	Questions	Answers
Page 4	Do you think the boy will get wet today?	Yes
	How do you know he will get wet?	Because it's raining outside.

Book 3 Brushing Teeth

	Questions	Answers
Page 1	What do you think the boy is going to do?	Brush his teeth
	How do you know he's going to brush his teeth?	Because he's holding his toothbrush and he is getting the toothpaste.
	What time of day is it?	Night-time
	How do you know it is night-time?	Because it's dark outside.
	What room of the house is this?	Bathroom
	How do you know it's the bathroom?	Because I can see a toilet, sink, etc.
Page 2	How many people do you think live in the boy's house?	Four
	How do you know this?	Because there are four toothbrushes altogether.
Page 3	How is the boy feeling?	Shocked
	How do you know he's shocked?	Because his eyes and mouth are wide open.

Book 4 Having a Haircut

	Questions	Answers
Page 1	Where is the boy?	In a hair salon/barbers
	How do you know he is in a hair salon/barbers?	Because the man is putting a cape on him and behind him there are mirrors, seats and trollies with hair salon things in them.
	How does the boy feel about having a haircut?	Sad
	How do you know he feels sad about it?	Because he looks sad.
	How does the hairdresser/barber feel about cutting the boy's hair?	Happy
	How do you know he's happy?	Because he is smiling.
	Is the hair salon/barbers busy?	No
	How do you know it's not busy?	Because there are no other customers.
Page 2	How does the boy feel when his hair is being shaved?	Uncomfortable/scared
	How do you know he is uncomfortable/scared?	Because his face looks uncomfortable.
	Do you think it's quiet or noisy in the hair salon right now?	Noisy
	How do you know it's noisy?	Because the electric razor is being used.
Page 3	How does the boy's hair feel?	Wet
	How do you know it's wet?	Because the hairdresser/barber is spraying it with water.
Page 5	How does the boy feel?	Happy
	How do you know he is happy?	Because he is smiling.

Book 4 Having a Haircut (continued)

	Questions	Answers
Page 6	How does the boy feel about his new haircut?	He likes it
	How do you know he likes it?	Because he has a big smile.
	Does the hairdresser/ barber like the haircut?	Yes
	How do you know he likes the haircut?	Because he is smiling.

Book 5 Walking the Dog

	Questions	Answers
Page 1	What is the weather like?	Sunny/warm
	How do you know it's warm?	Because the girl is wearing a t-shirt and shorts.
Page 2	Does the girl know the boy?	Yes
	How do you know she knows him?	Because she is waving at him.
Page 3	What does the girl want to do?	Cross the road.
	How do you know she wants to cross the road?	Because she is pressing the traffic light button.
Page 4	Is it safe to cross the road?	No
	How do you know it's not safe?	Because the traffic light is red.
Page 5	Is it safe to cross the road?	Yes
	How do you know it's safe?	Because the traffic light is green.

Book 5 Walking the Dog (continued)

	Questions	Answers
Page 6	Are the boy and girl happy to meet?	Yes
	How do you know they're happy to meet?	Because they are hugging each other.

Book 6 In the Bakery

	Questions	Answers
Page 1	What does the girl want?	A gingerbread man
	How do you know she wants a gingerbread man?	Because she's pointing to it.
Page 2	What does the boy want?	A gingerbread man
	How do you know he wants a gingerbread man?	Because he's pointing to it.
Page 3	How is the girl feeling?	Sad/upset
	How do you know she is sad/upset?	Because she is crying.
Page 4	What does the girl want now?	A pig biscuit
	How do you know she wants a pig biscuit?	Because she is pointing to it.
Page 6	How is the girl's mum feeling?	Happy
	How do you know she is happy?	Because she is smiling.

Book 7 In the Park

	Questions	Answers
Page 1	What is the weather like?	Warm/sunny
	How do you know it's warm/sunny?	Because the girls are wearing dresses.
Page 2	How is Mia feeling?	Shocked
	How do you know she is shocked?	Because her eyes and mouth are wide open.
Page 3	How is Mia feeling?	Sad
	How do you know she is sad?	Because she looks sad.
Page 4	How is Mia feeling now?	Very sad/upset
	How do you know she is feeling very sad/upset?	Because she is crying.
	What is Carmen doing?	Trying to make her feel better.
	How do you know she is trying to make her feel better?	She's put her hand on her shoulder.
Page 5 & 6	How are Mia and Carmen feeling?	Very happy
	How do you know they are very happy?	Because they have big smiles.

Book 8 Playing Hide and Seek

	Questions	Answers
Page 1	What do you think the girl and boy are playing?	Hide and seek
	How do you know they are playing hide and seek?	Because the boy is covering his eyes.
	Which room of the house do you think they're in?	Living room
	How do you know they're in the living room?	Because I can see a sofa.
	How many people do you think are in their family?	Four
	How do you know there are four people in their family?	Because in the family photo there are four people.
	Who do you think is older, the boy or the girl?	The boy
	Why do you think the boy is older?	Because he's taller than the girl.
Page 2	Does the boy know the girl is hiding behind the curtain?	No
	How do you know he doesn't know?	Because he didn't see her hiding there. His eyes are closed and his back is turned.
Page 6	Did they enjoy the game?	Yes
	How do you know they enjoyed it?	Because they're both smiling.

Book 9 At School

	Questions	Answers
Page 2	What does Tia want?	The felt pens
	How do you know she wants them?	Because she is pointing at them.
	Where in school are they?	A classroom
	How do you know they're in a classroom?	Because there's a table, drawers and cupboards.
Page 5	Does the teacher like Fiona's writing?	Yes
	How do you know she likes her writing?	Because she is smiling at her.
Page 6	Does the teacher like Tia's drawing?	Yes
	How do you know she likes her drawing?	Because she is smiling at her and giving her a thumbs up.

Book 10 Swimming

	Questions	Answers
Page 2	Do you think the boy is still learning to swim?	Yes
	How do you know he is still learning to swim?	Because he is wearing armbands.
Page 3	How is the boy feeling?	Scared
	How do you know he's scared?	Because he looks scared. He's got his hands on his cheeks.

Book 10 Swimming (continued)

	Questions	Answers
Page 4	What part of the boy's body is wet?	His feet
	How do you know his feet are wet?	Because they're in water.
Page 5	How does the boy's dad feel when the boy is swimming?	Happy
	How do you know he's happy?	Because he's smiling.
Page 6	How does the boy's dad feel?	Surprised
	How do you know he's surprised?	Because his mouth and eyes are wide open.

Topical conversation

As the books cover a range of familiar topics, they can be used as conversation starters and for building conversational skills. The key skills to work on are: asking and answering questions, commenting and staying on topic. Depending on the child's level of skill in this area, work could be done using structured scripts for those who require a guided approach, or flexible topic-related questions could be used with children who require less structure (i.e. children who have skills in asking and answering questions).

Below is an example of a short script:

Role	Theme: Play at home
You	What do you like to play at home?
Child	I like to play . . .
Child	What do you like to play at home?
You	I like to play . . .
You	Who do you play with?
Child	I play with . . .
Child	Who do you play with?
You	I play with . . .

A less structured approach would involve using a brainstorm with a range of questions on the topic:

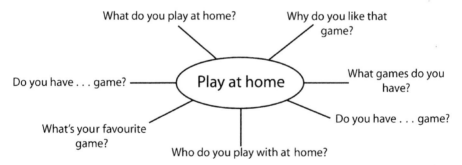

Below are points to consider before starting this section:

- For the structured approach, depending on the child's current level, you may start with just the first two steps and then work down scripts over time.

- Either a peer could have the conversation with the child, or you could yourself.

- You may need to tell the child what to say or give them suggestions for things they could say.

- You will need prior information about the child so that you can prompt them if you need to.

- A general tip for building conversational skills is to model statements that you would like the child to learn, so that they are exposed to ideas of what they could say and how to approach questions in future conversations.

Further reading

Baron-Cohen, S. (2001) 'Theory of mind in normal development and autism', *Prisme*, 34, pp. 174–83.

Calderdale and Huddersfield NHS Foundation Trust (2012) *Narrative Activity Pack: Support Pack for Schools*, Speech & Language Therapy Service.

McHugh, L., Bobarnac, A. & Reed, P. (2011) 'Brief report: teaching situation-based emotions to children with autistic spectrum disorder', *Journal of Autism and Developmental Disorders*, 41 pp. 1423–28.

Sundberg, M.L. (2008) *VB-MAPP, Verbal Behaviour Milestones Assessment and Placement Program*, AVB Press, Concord CA.

Westby, C. (2011) *Reading Between the Lines: Making Inferences*, online, www.speechpathology.com/articles/oelig-eading-between-lines-making-1526 (accessed November 2015).